MIX
Papier aus verantwortungsvollen Quellen
Paper from responsible sources
FSC® C105338

Kousalya Prabahar

Pediatric Upper Respiratory Tract Infection

Prescribing Pattern and Health Economics

Anchor Academic
Publishing

Prabahar, Kousalya: Pediatric Upper Respiratory Tract Infection. Prescribing Pattern and Health Economics, Hamburg, Anchor Academic Publishing 2017

Buch-ISBN: 978-3-96067-137-4
PDF-eBook-ISBN: 978-3-96067-637-9
Druck/Herstellung: Anchor Academic Publishing, Hamburg, 2017

Bibliografische Information der Deutschen Nationalbibliothek:
Die Deutsche Nationalbibliothek verzeichnet diese Publikation in der Deutschen Nationalbibliografie; detaillierte bibliografische Daten sind im Internet über http://dnb.d-nb.de abrufbar.

Bibliographical Information of the German National Library:
The German National Library lists this publication in the German National Bibliography. Detailed bibliographic data can be found at: http://dnb.d-nb.de

All rights reserved. This publication may not be reproduced, stored in a retrieval system or transmitted, in any form or by any means, electronic, mechanical, photocopying, recording or otherwise, without the prior permission of the publishers.

Das Werk einschließlich aller seiner Teile ist urheberrechtlich geschützt. Jede Verwertung außerhalb der Grenzen des Urheberrechtsgesetzes ist ohne Zustimmung des Verlages unzulässig und strafbar. Dies gilt insbesondere für Vervielfältigungen, Übersetzungen, Mikroverfilmungen und die Einspeicherung und Bearbeitung in elektronischen Systemen.

Die Wiedergabe von Gebrauchsnamen, Handelsnamen, Warenbezeichnungen usw. in diesem Werk berechtigt auch ohne besondere Kennzeichnung nicht zu der Annahme, dass solche Namen im Sinne der Warenzeichen- und Markenschutz-Gesetzgebung als frei zu betrachten wären und daher von jedermann benutzt werden dürften.

Die Informationen in diesem Werk wurden mit Sorgfalt erarbeitet. Dennoch können Fehler nicht vollständig ausgeschlossen werden und die Diplomica Verlag GmbH, die Autoren oder Übersetzer übernehmen keine juristische Verantwortung oder irgendeine Haftung für evtl. verbliebene fehlerhafte Angaben und deren Folgen.

Alle Rechte vorbehalten

© Anchor Academic Publishing, Imprint der Diplomica Verlag GmbH
Hermannstal 119k, 22119 Hamburg
http://www.diplomica-verlag.de, Hamburg 2017
Printed in Germany

CONTENTS

Chapter	Contents	Page No.
I	Abstract	1
II	Introduction	2
III	Literature review	13
IV	Aim and objectives	22
V	Methods	23
VI	Results	25
VII	Discussion	30
VIII	Conclusion	33
IX	Acknowledgments	34
X	References	35

LIST OF TABLES

No.	Table	Page No.
1	Age-wise distribution of children	25
2	Gender-wise distribution of children	26
3	Prescribing indicators among outpatients	27
4	List of drugs prescribed along with prescribing frequency	28
5	Health economic analysis of drugs prescribed	29

LIST OF FIGURES

No.	Figure	Page No.
1	Age-wise distribution of children	25
2	Gender-wise distribution of children	26

I. ABSTRACT

Background: It is necessary to ascertain current prescribing of antibiotics for upper respiratory tract infections (URTIs) to address potential overuse.

Objective: To analyse the current prescription patterns and the economics of drugs used in the treatment of URTI.

Methods: A prospective observational study was carried out in the out-patient department of paediatrics. Children of 1 month to 18 years, diagnosed with URTI by the physician were included in the study. The demographic details, drugs prescribed, dose, duration of therapy, cost of drug therapy were all noted from the outpatient record. The cost of individual drug was analysed and the health economic analysis of drugs were performed.

Results: The maximum number of children was in the age group of 1-5 years. The average number of drugs per encounter was found to be 2.01. Antihistamines were commonly prescribed and hence it cost more to the patients, followed by cough syrups.

Conclusion: Medical audit is effective in improvising the prescribing pattern. Long-term interventional studies are needed to enhance the rational prescribing.

KEY WORDS: Paediatrics, economics, URTI.

II. INTRODUCTION

Upper respiratory tract infection (URTI) non-specifically describes acute infections involving nose, paranasal sinuses, pharynx, larynx, trachea and bronchi caused by many viruses, mainly rhinovirus.[1,2] A small percentage of cases (0.5–10%) are sometimes accompanied by bacterial infections.[3]

Prescribing antibiotics routinely for URTIs is not justified as they have limited clinical efficacy. However, they are more commonly prescribed in situations where they are not indicated such as in infections with bacterial uncertainty or uncertain viral etiology.[4-7]

The evolving public health threat of antimicrobial resistance (AMR) is driven by both appropriate and inappropriate use of anti-infective medicines for human and animal health and food production, together with inadequate measures to control the spread of infections. Recognizing the public health crisis due to AMR, several nations, international agencies, and many other organizations worldwide have taken action to counteract it through strategies applied in the relevant sectors. Several World Health Assembly resolutions have called for action on specific health aspects related to AMR, and the World Health Organization published its global strategy to contain AMR in 2001.[8]

On World Health Day (WHD) 2011, in a six-point policy package, countries were called upon to:

(1) Commit to a comprehensive, financed national plan with accountability and civil society engagement

(2) Strengthen surveillance and laboratory capacity

(3) Ensure uninterrupted access to essential medicines of assured quality

(4) Regulate and promote rational use of medicines in animal husbandry and to ensure proper patient care

(5) Enhance infection prevention and control

(6) Foster innovations and research and development of new tools.[9]

Paediatric respiratory tract infections are one of the most common reasons for physician visits and hospitalisation, and are associated with significant morbidity and mortality. Respiratory infections are common and frequent diseases and present one of the major complaints in children and adolescents. The role of physicians and other healthcare providers has expanded from merely treating disease to implementing measures aimed at health maintenance and disease prevention.[10]

Respiratory infections (RI), mainly involving the upper airways, are common in children and their recurrence constitutes a demanding challenge for the paediatricians. There are many children suffering from so-called recurrent respiratory infections (RRI). The child with recurrent respiratory infections presents a difficult diagnostic challenge. It is necessary to discriminate between those with simply-managed cause for their symptoms such as recurrent viral infections or asthma, from the children with more serious underlying pathology such as bronchiectasis or immune dysfunction. Many different disorders present this way, including cystic fibrosis, various immunodeficiency syndromes, congenital anomalies of respiratory tract, but in some children lung damage could follow a single severe pneumonia or can be the consequence of the inhalation of food or foreign body.[11]

According to the epidemiological studies it was estimated that around 6% of the children younger than 6 years of age present RRI. In developed countries, up to 25% of children aged < 1 year and 18% of children aged 1-4 years, experience RRI.[10] Moreover, ENT infections represent the most frequent pathologies in children aged from 6 months to 6 years. Although the etiologic agents responsible for RRI are not always readily identifiable, viral agents are typically the main cause.

The real task for the paediatricians is to discriminate the normal children with high respiratory infections frequency related to an augmented exposure to environmental risk factors from the children affected by other underlying pathological conditions (immunological or not), predisposing to infectious respiratory diseases.[12] Usually, the children with RRI are not affected by severe alterations and RRI represent essentially the consequence of an increased exposure to infectious agents due to environmental factors during the first years of life.[13]

In the clinical practice, most of the children suffer from the recurrent infections of the upper airways, but in approximately 10-30%, the lower tract is also affected. There are two peaks of the incidence of RRI:[11]

- 6-12 months of age - after consumption of the maternal passively transferred immunoglobulins with concomitant postponed synthesis of own antibodies
- the involvement of the child in to the group of children at nursery or school.

Upper respiratory infections are common but are unlikely to indicate an underlying medical condition when they occur in isolation. When evaluating the patients with recurrent infections, it is reasonable to use acronym SPUR (severe, persistent, unusual, recurrent) to prompt appropriate investigations for underlying causes. Children with RRI have the course of the airway infections (feature, severity and duration) similar to those presented by children with "normal" incidence of respiratory infections. The frequency of RI in children with RRI shows typical seasonality with the highest rate during autumn and winter.[13] Typically, these children are not affected by the recurrent infections of the other systems (gastrointestinal tract, central nervous system, uro-genital tract or skin). While most children with recurrent infection have a normal immunity, it is important to recognize the child with an underlying primary immunodeficiency and investigate and treat appropriately and not over-investigate normal children.[14]

RRI are a common problem mainly in preschool age, usually due to the presence of unfavourable environmental conditions, including early socialization, as well as the immaturity and inexperience of the immune system.[15] In infancy and early childhood, the immune system encounters antigens for the first time, mounting immune responses and acquiring memory. Young children mix with other children in families or nursery and are exposed to many pathogens and therefore there are more vulnerable to infection and recurrent infections are common.[14] Many of the children are simply having the repeated viral upper respiratory tract infections that are a normal part of growing up. In others, the symptoms are the first manifestations of asthma.

If there is a history of persistent or recurrent pneumonia with or without chronic sputum production, it is indicating more severe pathology.[11] RRI initially occur as a viral respiratory tract infection, but bacterial growth is demonstrated in 60% of patients with symptoms of an upper respiratory tract infection of at least 10 days duration.[16,17] The children with prolonged or recurrent respiratory illnesses most often have a series of infections rather than persistent infection with one virus strain.[18] Some children experience considerable morbidity as a result of RRI and receive repeated courses of antibacterials that are not effective against viral infectious agents and can increase bacterial resistance.[19] Hence, URTIs is a major burden to the healthcare systems, especially when inappropriate antibiotic treatment leads to increased antibiotic resistance.[20]

Infections of the Upper Respiratory Tract (URT) are the most commonly encountered illness of childhood[21] and one of the main reasons for pediatric consultations.[22,23] More than 200 viruses can cause upper respiratory tract infections (URTIs). Acute respiratory infection accounts for 20-40% of outpatient in Pediatrics.[24] The emergence of bacterial resistance to antimicrobials is a growing concern all over the world.[25] The relationship between the use of antibiotics and the development of resistance is confirmed by various studies.[26,27] Antibiotics are commonly used for treating of upper respiratory tract infections, although viruses cause most of URTIs.[28]

Anti Microbial Agents (AMAs) are the most frequently used drug and it is misused more commonly compared to all other drugs. The inevitable consequence of the common use of AMAs has been the emergence of antibiotic resistant pathogens, fuelling an ever increasing need for new drugs. Decreasing inappropriate antibiotic use is the best way to reduce or control resistance. Eventhough there are increased awareness about the harmful effects of antibiotic misuse, over prescribing remains widespread. It mainly occurs by patient demand, time pressure on clinicians and diagnostic uncertainty. Appropriate selection of AMAs for treating infectious diseases requires clinical judgment of disease and the drugs. The bacterial infection should be identified before treatment and should be initiated whenever possible. To initiate right choice of empirical antibiotic therapy, knowledge on the most likely infecting microorganism and their susceptibilities to antimicrobial drugs is essential.[29]

The bacterial agents that are resistant to antibiotics are of greatest concern. These resistance are mainly due to common and inappropriate antibiotic therapy for children with upper respiratory tract illnesses. Approximately three fourths of all outpatient antibiotic prescriptions given to children are for upper respiratory tract conditions mainly viral infections, bronchitis, pharyngitis, sinusitis, and otitis media. To reduce and look into this problem, the Centers for Disease Control and Prevention (CDC) and the American Academy of Pediatrics published "The Principles of Judicious Use of Antimicrobial Agents for Pediatric Upper Respiratory Tract Infections".[5] This document focuses on reducing the antibiotic usage for such conditions that do not respond to them and promoting the use of narrow- rather than broad-spectrum antibiotics.

Respiratory infections are the major reason for prescribing antibiotics in paediatrics. According to the 1992 National Ambulatory Medical Care Survey

(NAMCS) in the United States, acute otitis media was the most common diagnosis for which antibiotics were prescribed (30%), followed by upper respiratory tract infection (URTI), pharyngitis and bronchitis (12%, 10% and 9%, respectively).[30] Inappropriate prescription of antibiotics can lead to the emergence of bacterial resistance, an increase in adverse drug effects and high pressure on financial burden.

In November 2013, The American Academy of Pediatrics released a set of three basic principles for the effective use of antibiotics to treat pediatric URIs, including acute otitis media, acute bacterial sinusitis, and streptococcal pharyngitis.[31,32] The principles are as follows:

- Accurate diagnosis of a bacterial infection;
- Consideration of the risks vs benefits of antibiotic treatment; and
- Implementation of judicious prescribing strategies, including selection of the most effective antibiotic, prescription of an appropriate dose, and treating for the shortest possible duration.

These principles will help healthcare providers distinguish bacterial infections from viral infections.

Medical audit looks into the standards of medical treatment at all levels of the healthcare delivery system.[32] Prescribing pattern study is a part of the medical audit and it monitors, evaluates and suggest modifications in prescribing practices to make medical care rational and cost-effective.

The CDC in collaboration with the American Academy of Paediatrics (AAP) recommends stringent diagnostic criteria for URTIs to avoid misdiagnosis and inappropriate antibiotic prescriptions. Antibiotic treatment is helpful to children only if symptoms persist for 10-14 days without any improvement.[33]

New drugs and new modes of treatment are constantly being introduced. The medical care's quality should be judicially implemented, appropriate, safe, effective and economic. "Good" prescribing is a complex balance between various conflicting factors.[34]

Recommendations

The following recommendations can be made regarding the use of antimicrobials in RTIs of all age groups:

1) The prescriber should be aware of the costs of the drugs they are prescribing. In some studies from USA has been reported that many prescribes have rather poor knowledge of the drug they are prescribing. Institutional and independent educational training programmed can achieve this. Institutions should encourage practioners to examine their own prescription and to compare the cost effectiveness of alternative therapeutic regimens.

2) Appropriate information about the antimicrobials should be available to the public at all levels

3) Public should be made aware that antimicrobials are strong drugs having side effects and drug interactions. It should not be use for common cold right away because in most case they are of viral origin and antimicrobial are of no use in viral infections, therefore, should not be taken on their own unless prescribed by a doctor. Old prescriptions for any RTIs should not be used for new and recent illnesses. The patient should not discuss their disease with neighbours, friends and chemists to avoid improper use of drugs in general and antimicrobials in particular. National awareness programmes can achieve this and massive educations programmes especially at school levels.

4) Prescriber should be encouraged to use minimum of drug regimen without sacrificing the efficacy of treatment, or therapeutic benefits.

5) Effective antimicrobial national policy should be implemented.

6) Prescription of expensive drugs should be discouraged.

This study attempts to analyze the current prescription patterns and the economics of drugs used in the treatment of URTI. Findings of this study are expected to provide relevant and useful feedback to pediatricians and general practitioners.

III. LITERATURE REVIEW

Indian Scenario

Antibiotic prescriptions were inappropriate in acute self-limiting upper respiratory tract infection. Antibiotics are over prescribed for paediatric URTIs. Doctors should be educated on more appropriate and cost effective prescribing.[35]

Non-specific URTI is the most common condition among the respiratory tract infection (RTI). Polypharmacy is prevalent in the OPD of paediatrics. The prescribers should be trained as per the guideline for the management of RTI. The parents and the physicians should be sensitized that antibiotics, cough syrup, antihistamines are not always helpful in the treatment of RTI and vitamins and minerals, digestive enzymes and liver syrup have no role in the treatment of RTIs. An essential drug list for a hospital and problem-based basic training in pharmacotherapy should be advocated. Availability, accessibility, and affordability of drugs of good quality; drug information centres; drug use evaluation and drug bulletins should be provided to the users and the prescribers. "Hospital May Be Hazardous To Health". So to escape medication errors constant scrutiny of medications and prescribing and dispensing must be done regularly.[36]

In India, approximately 35% of population comprises of children below 12 years which is a very large number. Hence, provision of good health care to them indirectly reflects on the healthcare set-up of the country.[37] Rational drug utilization needs training of health professionals in treatment guidelines and prescriber education to ensure appropriate therapy. There is a need for education of both parents and doctors regarding the limited help of antibiotics or other drugs for this self-limiting condition. Regular studies such as this are the need of the hour to study drug prescribing practices so that appropriate feedback and awareness is generated. Moreover, the prescribing patterns reflects the ability of prescriber in terms of choosing such drugs which are accessible, affordable, safe, effective and give maximum benefit to patients. Thus, to ensure the rationality of drug prescription time to time monitoring, evaluation is absolutely essential as changes in health related behaviour usually take longer to achieve.[38]

Misuse/overuse of antibiotics is a major public health issue that affects both the community as well as the individuals. Unless the infection in children prove to be bacterial, use of antibiotics for URTIs is inappropriate. Antibiotic misuse, especially in pediatrics could lead to bacterial resistance and other undesirable side effects. The minimal antibiotic and injections usage reflects judicious choice on the part of the prescriber. This serves as an evidence based study on the rational use of antibiotic in URTIs in pediatric outpatient clinic.[39]

Inappropriate use of antibiotics for treating RTIs which are mainly due to virus and do not require antibiotic treatment are practiced. Results warrant interventional strategies to promote rational use of antibiotics and to decrease the emerging antibiotic resistance. Standard treatment guidelines for the treatment of respiratory tract infections should developed and implemented.[40]

Infections of the upper respiratory tract including nose, the para nasal sinuses, adenoids, tonsils, nasopharynx and eustachian tube is the most frequently occurring illness of childhood. Most instances of URTI are of viral origin and resolve spontaneously. Antibiotic treatment is needed only if symptoms persist for 10-14 days. There is a need of rational prescription of medicines to minimize medicinal error in children. The pattern of prescriptions in URTI in children aged 1 to 14 years were analyzed and evaluated for the rationality of drug usage. The data from the outpatient record of each patient was collected in a separate proforma and subjected to descriptive statistical analysis using Microsoft Excel. The study included only one prescription per patient. Utilization of different classes of drugs as well as individual drug was analyzed and presented as percentage. Remedial measures were suggested to avoid erroneous prescriptions.[34]

Prescribing by generic name should be encouraged. Use of parenteral antibiotics was high and route conversion programmes should be instituted. Use of antibiotics for predominantly viral infections should be reduced. Treatment guidelines for common conditions should be formulated.[41]

Upper respiratory tract infections constitute 87.5% of the respiratory infections. Majority of upper respiratory tract infections are mainly caused by viruses. In many circumstances, common cold is caused by viruses and it does not require an antimicrobial agent unless there are complications. Most of the URTIs resolve automatically without antimicrobials.[24]

In rural area, mothers had very poor information regarding the mode of transmission, diagnosis, available treatments, treatment utilization and URTI complications and low utilization of basic health services from government hospitals. Health education can change the health care attitude and behaviors of parents to take care of URTIs. The educational information activities and the female literacy level should be strengthened to control and prevent URTI. Proper training of health care workers in identification and timely management of URTI is essential.[42]

Global Perspective

Physicians are slowly improving their antibiotic prescribing patterns but the use of inappropriate antibiotics is still common. Despite modest improvements demonstrated by a review of the National Ambulatory Medical Care Survey data, inappropriate antibiotic use is still common. Almost half of patients with URTIs received antibiotics even though these conditions are known to be of viral origin. Even in conditions like sinusitis and otitis media, for which antibiotic therapy is appropriate, an inappropriate antibiotic is used more than 10% of the time. Interventions to improve the prescribing of antibiotics should focus on changing treatment patterns for both URTIs and bronchitis. The interventions should be aimed at all types of physicians and also directed toward parents and patients to dampen their enthusiasm for antibiotics.[43]

Antibiotic resistance is associated with prior receipt of antibiotics. An analysis of linked computerized databases for physician visits and antibiotic prescriptions was used to examine antibiotic prescribing for different respiratory infections in preschool children in Canada. Antibiotics were prescribed to 49% of children with upper respiratory tract infection, 18% with nasopharyngitis, 78% with pharyngitis or tonsillitis, 32% with serous otitis media, 80% with acute otitis media, 61% with sinusitis, 44% with acute laryngitis or tracheitis, and 24% with influenza. Acute otitis media accounted for 33% of all visits and

39% of all antibiotic prescriptions. The estimated Canadian dollar cost of overprescribing was $423,693, or 49% of the total cost of antibiotics ($859,893) used in this group. This population-based study confirms antibiotic overprescribing in Canada.[44]

Although overuse of antibiotics in children has been well documented, relatively little information is known about provider and facility characteristics associated with this prescribing practice. This study was done to evaluate the differences in overuse of antibiotics among staff physicians and resident/interns (housestaff [HS]) who work in hospital-based outpatient clinics. Antibiotic prescribing in the context of an outpatient visit for a diagnosis suggestive of a viral respiratory tract illness occurs more commonly among staff physicians than trainees and among staff physicians more commonly in nonteaching compared with teaching institutions.[45]

The proper and correct use of antimicrobial is an utmost necessity of current situation in today's world. The emerging antimicrobial resistance is a global problem directly related to inappropriate use. This study has shown that antimicrobial is widely prescribed for RTI in all the cases. Indiscriminate usage of antibiotics could increase the cost of therapy, incidence of adverse drug reaction, and increase in the rate of emergence of bacterial resistance.[46]

Antibiotics misuse/overuse is an important public health issue that affects the community and the individual. Using antibiotics to treat children from upper respiratory tract infections is evidently inappropriate unless the infection was proven to be bacterial. This misuse of antibiotics, especially in children, will increase the risk of developing bacterial resistance which emphasis on the need to discover the contributing factors to this overuse of antibiotics. Factors influencing the misuse/overuse of antibiotics in the literature include:

(1) psychosocial factors, such as: behaviors, beliefs, and attitudes (e.g., self-medication & over-the-counter medication),

(2) parents pressure, often documented by doctors,

(3) demographic characteristics (e.g., socio-economic status, education levels) and

(4) lack of health education.

Discovering the factors affecting the misuse/overuse of antibiotics, whether they are patients'/ parents'-related or doctors'-related could assist in the development and implementation of a well-designed methodological intervention protocol that can lead to a decrease in antibiotics use.

Interventions that could lead to the reduction in antibiotics overuse may include: (1) health education campaigns, professional education as well as public awareness campaigns are evidently effective in the reduction of the unnecessary use of antibiotics in children with upper respiratory tract infections.

(2) Doctor-patients interactions, where the patient/parent gets involved in the decision making process with the doctor. And/or

(3) policy change, such as: implementing a new policy for delaying antibiotics prescription for 48 hours which will give the self-limiting conditions to time to heal without the use of medications.

Choosing the best intervention protocol relays on discovering the most influencing factor(s) associated with this overuse.[47]

An algorithm for treating common childhood conditions seen at this centre needs to be developed and circulated among doctors attending to these children. Having a handbook of the national formulary for easy referencing before prescribing will go a long way to minimising inappropriate drug prescriptions. Also, continuous medical education with focus on rational drug use and evidence based medicine should form part of the programme of the hospital.[48]

A targeted educational intervention can improve antibiotic prescription practices for respiratory infections in children and decrease unnecessary antibiotic use. Such studies can also pinpoint areas that require further attention. The optimal method of education is still unclear, but it should probably include ongoing campaigns for both physicians and parents at local and nationwide levels. Further investigation is needed to identify areas that require more attention, such as sinusitis in our study, and to determine the long-term effect of such interventions.[49]

The first population-based community study of RTI in Inuit children <2 years of age based on active surveillance showed an overall high occurrence of the disease. A total of 41.6% of days were spent with symptoms of respiratory tract infections, and the incidence of new episodes of acute respiratory infection was 2.5 per 100 days at risk. Of all episodes, 65% caused activity restriction, and 40% caused contact with the health center. The prevalence of this disease calls for intervention programs, and further studies are needed to elucidate risk factors that may allow for specific interventions.[50]

Paediatric recurrent RTIs represent a huge global health burden, resulting in much morbidity and mortality in children. Moreover, they contribute greatly to socioeconomic costs in the form of absenteeism from work of parents as well as visits to the general practitioner. Antibacterial treatments are often prescribed in this population; however, they have limited efficacy and, more importantly, increase the level of antibiotic resistance around the world. Preventive measures are therefore an essential alternative for the management of this disease and help reduce the risk of developing respiratory infections. At present, many practitioners still fail to employ prevention strategies in children with recurrent RTIs. Currently there are several immunostimulants approved for use in treating recurrent RTIs and future trends will look to using and developing these more, making them available to a greater number of nations – particularly within developing countries that see higher child mortality rates from these diseases.[51]

IV. AIM AND OBJECTIVES

AIM:

To study the prescribing pattern and health economics in URTI in the paediatric out-patient department with respect to antibiotics in a tertiary care teaching hospital.

OBJECTIVES:

- ❖ To study the prescribing patterns in URTI in the paediatric out-patient department
- ❖ To study health economics in URTI in the paediatric out-patient department

V. METHODS

STUDY SITE	: Out-patient department of paediatrics, a tertiary care teaching hospital
STUDY PERIOD	: 2 months
STUDY DESIGN	: Prospective observational study
INCLUSION CRITERIA	: Children 1month to 18years, diagnosed with URTI by the physician.
EXCLUSION CRITERIA	: Children with lower respiratory infections/ wheeze/gastro intestinal symptoms and pre-existing symptoms.

Children with co-morbid conditions like

-Heart disease

-Asthma

-Kidney disease

-Liver disease

The data for children with diagnosis of URTI from the out- patient record of each patient was collected in a proforma, after getting approval from the Research and Ethics Committee.

The demographic details, drugs prescribed, dose, duration of therapy, cost of drug therapy were all recorded and the data was analysed. The cost of individual drug was analysed and the health economic analysis of drugs were performed.

Statistical Analysis

All the data were entered in Microsoft Excel and the mean and standard deviation was calculated. The results were entered in frequency and percentage.

VI. RESULTS

During our study period, 150 prescriptions were analyzed. The maximum number of children was in the age group of 1-5 years (n = 81, 54%), followed by less than 1 year (n = 48, 32%). No children were found in the age group of more than 10 years (Table 1, Figure 1).

Table 1: Age-wise distribution of children

Age (In years)	n	%
<1	48	32
1 – 5	81	54
5 – 10	21	14
10 – 18	-	-

Figure 1: Age-wise distribution of children

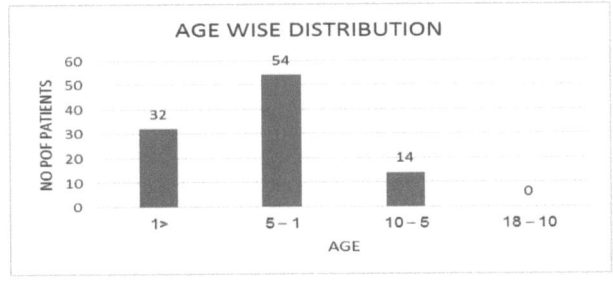

Male children were found to be predominant (n = 88, 58.7%) (Table 2, Figure 2).

Table 2: Gender-wise distribution of children

SEX	n	%
Male	88	58.66
Female	62	41.33

Figure 2: Gender-wise distribution of children

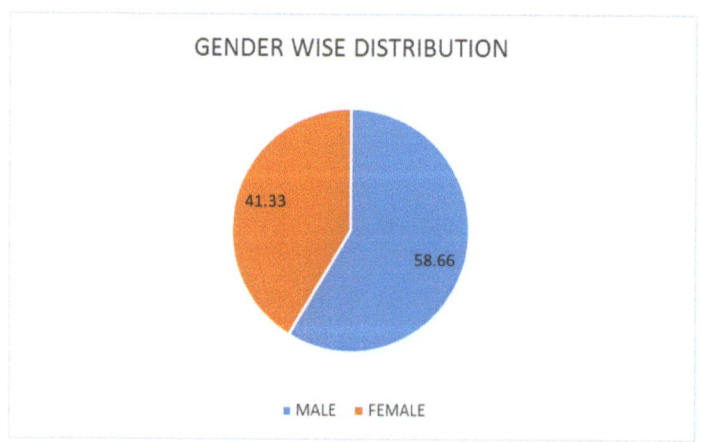

The prescribing indicators among the children was given in table 3. The average number of drugs per encounter was found to be 2.01.

Table 3: Prescribing indicators among outpatients

Parameter	Number
Total number of patients prescriptions analyzed	150
Total number of drugs prescribed	302
Average number of drugs per encounter	2.01

The list of drugs prescribed to the children were grouped into analgesics and antipyretics, antihistamines, antibiotics, cough syrups and miscellaneous. The prescribed drugs and the prescribing frequency were depicted in table 4. This table indicates that antibiotics were used minimally in children. Antihistamines were prescribed commonly.

Table 4: List of drugs prescribed along with prescribing frequency

Drug Categories	Prescriptions	
	n = 302	%
Analgesics & Antipyretics	35	11.59
Antihistamines	129	42.72
Antibiotics	10	3.31
Cough syrups	99	32.78
Miscellaneous	29	9.60

The cost of individual drug was analysed and the health economic analysis of drugs prescribed was given in table 5. The drugs were grouped into the same as in table 4. Antihistamines cost more compared to other drugs followed by cough syrups.

Table 5: Health economic analysis of drugs prescribed

Drug group	Average cost of the drug per dose per child (INR)
Analgesics & Antipyretics	0.54
Antihistamines	1.82
Antibiotics	0.16
Cough syrups	1.20
Miscellaneous	0.19

VII. DISCUSSION

Audit studies are methods of improving job satisfaction of the health care professionals and it serves as a means of education for them, rather than being considered as a threat or another bureaucratic burden. In our study, the majority of children were in the age group of 1-5 years. This was similar to the study conducted by Nandimath and Ahuja, 2012.[34]

The average number of drugs per prescription was 2.01. The lower number of drugs noted is a welcome sign and needs to be encouraged. There may be a rise in adherence, minimal cost of therapy and minimized risk of drug interactions when lesser number of drugs is prescribed.

In our study, most of the drugs were prescribed by brand name. This was similar to the study conducted by Oshikoya et al., 2006.[48]

In this study, antihistamines were found to be the most frequently prescribed drugs. As the under five group constituted the major proportion of patients with URTI for whom antihistamine was prescribed, this implies that a huge amount of costly drugs were unnecessarily prescribed. Similar result was observed in various studies.[34,41]

Cough syrups play an important role in the prescriptions. Antibiotics were used only for 3.31% of children. It was similar to the study conducted by Shankar et al., 2006.[41]

Antibiotic resistance is the most common emerging problem in the health care field. Inappropriate and abundant use of antibiotics is a major contributor to this ever-growing problem. The majority of childhood URTI is caused by viruses which do not require antibiotics. Hence the minimal use of antibiotics show a positive sign of rational prescribing. Moreover, pescribing an antibiotic or an antihistamine for URTI may reinforce the parent's belief in the necessity of such treatment every time the child develops such symptoms. The decreased prescribing of antibiotics cannot be linked only to our intervention. Many publications in the medical literature and in the public media have alerted physicians to the unwanted effects of antibiotic overuse and have led to a worldwide decrease in antibiotic prescription for paediatrics.

On an average, two drugs was prescribed per child. There was no drug duplication in any prescription.

Most of drugs were not prescribed from essential drug list. The low rate of prescribing of essential drugs is a matter of concern. The use of anti-histamine, cetirizine which is not on the essential drug list may be a contributory factor for increased cost.

Irrational prescribing is a habit that is difficult to cure.[52] However, prevention is possible by short problem based training course in pharmacotherapy and rational use focused workshop interventions.[53] It is essential to increase doctors' awareness of the lack of proven benefits, the definitive cost and side effects of many prescriptions for the self-limiting illness. Doctors should be trained and educated on the most appropriate and cost effective use of antibiotics. There have been many forum aimed at altering physician's prescribing behaviour. These have included audit studies, group discussions and feedback, introduction of hospital formulary and guidelines for antibiotics. The benefits of the intervention studies, namely the use of fewer and cheaper prescriptions are shown to disappear overtime, which suggests the need for repeating the intervention at frequent intervals. Rational prescribing messages should be promoted at national and local medical meetings.

VIII. CONCLUSION

Medical audit is effective in improvising the prescribing pattern. Long-term interventional studies are needed to enhance the rational prescribing.

IX. ACKNOWLEDGMENTS

I extend my sincere thanks to the publisher, for their dedication in bringing this book and making my dream come true.

X. REFERENCES

1. Heikkinen T, Järvinen A. The common cold. Lancet 2003;361(9351): 51-9.

2. Lau SK, Yip CC, Tsoi HW, et al. Clinical features and complete genome characterization of a distinct human rhinovirus (HRV) genetic cluster, probably representing a previously undetected HRV species, human rhinovirus-C, associated with acute respiratory illness in children. J Clin Microbiol 2007;45(11):3655-64.

3. Mossad SB. Upper respiratory tract infections, 2011. Available from: www.clevelandclinicmeded.com/medicalpubs/diseasemanagement/inf ectious-disease/upper-respiratory-tract-infection/Default.htm. [Last accessed March 2017].

4. Gonzales R, Bartlett JG, Besser RE, et al. Principles of appropriate antibiotic use for treatment of acute respiratory tract infections in adults: background, specific aims, and methods. Ann Intern Med 2001;134(6):479-86.

5. Dowell SF, Marcy M, Phillips WR, Gerber MA, Shwartz B. Principles of judicious use of antimicrobial agents for pediatric upper respiratory tract infections. Pediatrics 1998;101(1):163-5.

6. Kumarasamy KK, Toleman MA, Walsh TR, et al. Emergence of a new antibiotic resistance mechanism in India, Pakistan, and the UK: a

molecular, biological, and epidemiological study. Lancet Infect Dis 2010;10(9):597-602.

7. World Health Organization. The evolving threat of antimicrobial resistance: options for action, 2012. Available from: http://whqlibdoc.who.int/publications/2012/9789241503181_eng.pdf [Last accessed March 2017].

8. WHO Global Strategy for Containment of Antimicrobial Resistance. Geneva, World Health Organization, WHO/CDS/CSR/DRS/2001.2, 2001. Available from:

http://www.who.int/csr/resources/publications/drugresist/en/EGlobal_Strat.pdf [Last accessed March 2017].

9. World Health Day 2011: Policy briefs. Geneva, World Health Organization, 2011. Available from: http://www.who.int/ world-health-day/2011/policybriefs/en/index.html [Last accessed March 2017].

10. Bellanti JA. Recurrent respiratory tract infections in paediatric patients. Drugs 1997;54(1):1-4.

11. Couriel J. Assessment of the child with recurrent chest infections. Br Med Bull 2002;61:115-32.

12. de Martino M, Balloti S. The child with recurrent respiratory infections: normal or not? Pediatr Allergy Immunol 2007;18(18):13-8.

13. Arden KE, McErlean P, Nissen MD, Sloots TP, Mackay IM. Frequent detection of human rhinoviruses, paramyxoviruses, coronaviruses, and bocavirus during acute respiratory tract infections. J Med Virol 2006;78(9):1232-40.

14. Slatter MA, Gennery AR. Clinical immunology review series: an approach to the patient with recurrent infections in childhood. Clin Exp Immunol 2008;152(3):389-96.

15. Dellepiane RM, Pavesi P, Patria MF, Laicini E, Di Landro G, Pietrogrande MC. Atopy in preschool Italian children with recurrent respiratory infections. Pediatr Med Chir 2009;31(4):161-4.

16. Kowalska M, Kowalska H, Zawadzka-Glos L, et al. Dysfunction of peripheral blood granulocyte oxidative metabolism in children with recurrent upper respiratory tract infections. Int J Pediatr Otorhinolaryngol 2003;67(4):365-71.

17. Salami A, Dellepiane M, Crippa B, et al. Sulphurous water inhalations in the prophylaxis of recurrent upper respiratory tract infections. Int J Pediatr Otorhinolaryngol 2008;72(11):1717-22.

18. Jartti T, Lee WM, Pappas T, Evans M, Lemanske RF, Gern JE. Serial viral infections in infants with recurrent respiratory illnesses. Eur Respir J 2008;32(2):314-20.

19. Bousquet J, Fiocchi A. Prevention of recurrent respiratory tract infections in children using a ribosomal immunotherapeutic agent: a clinical review. Pediatr Drugs 2006;8(4):235-43.

20. Schlossberg D. Clinical approach to antibiotic failure. Med Clin North Am 2006;90(6):1265-77.

21. Herendeen NE, Szilagy PG. Infections of the upper respiratory tract. Nelson Textbook of Pediatrics, Edn 16, Philadelphia, W B Saunders Company, 2000, p.1261-6.

22. Teng CL, Shajahan Y, Khoo EM, Nurjahan I, Leong KC, Yap TG. The management of upper respiratory tract infections. Med J Malaysia 2001;56(2):260-6.

23. Mlynarczyk G, Mlynarczyk A, Jeljaszewicz J. Epidemiological aspects of antibiotic resistance in respiratory pathogens. Int J Antimicrob Agents 2001;18(6):497-502.

24. Jain N, Lodha R, Kabra SK. Upper respiratory tract infections. Indian J Pediatr 2001;68(12):1135-8.

25. Spellberg B, Guidos R, Gilbert D, et al. The epidemic of antibiotic-resistant infections: a call to action for the medical community from the Infectious Diseases Society of America. Clin Infect Dis 2008;46(2):155–64.

26. Costelloe C, Metcalfe C, Lovering A, Mant D, Hay AD. Effect of antibiotic prescribing in primary care on antimicrobial resistance in

individual patients: systematic review and meta-analysis. BMJ 2010;340:c2096.

27. Yagupsky P. Selection of antibiotic-resistant pathogens in the community. Pediatr Infect Dis J 2006;25(10):974–6.

28. Earnshaw S, Monnet DL, Duncan B, et al. European Antibiotic Awareness Day, 2008 - The first Europe-wide public information campaign on prudent antibiotic use: methods and survey of activities in participating countries. Euro Surveill 2009;14(30):19280.

29. Chambers HF. General principles of antimicrobial therapy. Goodman & Gilman's The Pharmacological Basis of Therapeutics, Edn 11, New York, McGraw-Hill, 2006, p.1095-110.

30. McCaig LF, Hughes JM. Trends in antimicrobial drug prescribing among office-based physicians in United States. JAMA 1995;273(3):214–9.

31. Hersh AL, Jackson MA, Hicks LA, American Academy of Pediatrics Committee on Infectious Diseases. Principles of judicious antibiotic prescribing for upper respiratory tract infections in pediatrics. Pediatrics 2013;132(6):1146-54.

32. Gupta N, Gupta D, Sharma D, Garg SK, Bhargava VK. Auditing of prescriptions to study utilization of antimicrobials in a tertiary hospital. Indian J Pharmacol 1997;29:411-5.

33. Rosentein N, Phillips WR, Gerber MA, Marcy MS, Schwartz B, Dowell SF. The common cold - principles of judicious use of antimicrobial agents. Pediatrics 1998;101(1):181-4.

34. Nandimath MK, Ahuja S. Drug prescribing pattern in upper respiratory tract infection in children aged 1 - 14 years. Int J Pharma Bio Sci 2012;3(1):299-308.

35. Joseph N, Bharathi DR, Sreenivasa B, Nataraj GR, George N, Safdar M. Prescribing pattern of drugs in upper respiratory tract infections in pediatric out patients. Int J Contemp Pediatr 2016;3(3):1006-8.

36. Bikash G, Devarsi C, Daisy P, Deka A. Drug prescribing pattern in respiratory tract infection in children aged 1 to 12 years at outpatient department at Silchar Medical College and Hospital, Assam, India. J Pharm Biomed Sci 2016;6(10): 537–45.

37. Park K. Preventive Medicine in Obstetrics, Paediatrics and Geriartics. Park's textbook of Preventive and Social Medicine, 23rd edition, 2015.

38. Sharma S, Agarwal G. A study on drug prescribing pattern in upper respiratory tract infections among children aged 1-12 years. Int J Basic Clin Pharmacol 2016;5(2):406-10.

39. Tiwari P, Ahlawat R, Gupta G. Prescription practice in patients of upper respiratory tract infection at a pediatric outpatient clinic in Punjab. Indian Journal of Pharmacy Practice 2014;7(2):26-32.

individual patients: systematic review and meta-analysis. BMJ 2010;340:c2096.

27. Yagupsky P. Selection of antibiotic-resistant pathogens in the community. Pediatr Infect Dis J 2006;25(10):974–6.

28. Earnshaw S, Monnet DL, Duncan B, et al. European Antibiotic Awareness Day, 2008 - The first Europe-wide public information campaign on prudent antibiotic use: methods and survey of activities in participating countries. Euro Surveill 2009;14(30):19280.

29. Chambers HF. General principles of antimicrobial therapy. Goodman & Gilman's The Pharmacological Basis of Therapeutics, Edn 11, New York, McGraw-Hill, 2006, p.1095-110.

30. McCaig LF, Hughes JM. Trends in antimicrobial drug prescribing among office-based physicians in United States. JAMA 1995;273(3):214–9.

31. Hersh AL, Jackson MA, Hicks LA, American Academy of Pediatrics Committee on Infectious Diseases. Principles of judicious antibiotic prescribing for upper respiratory tract infections in pediatrics. Pediatrics 2013;132(6):1146-54.

32. Gupta N, Gupta D, Sharma D, Garg SK, Bhargava VK. Auditing of prescriptions to study utilization of antimicrobials in a tertiary hospital. Indian J Pharmacol 1997;29:411-5.

33. Rosentein N, Phillips WR, Gerber MA, Marcy MS, Schwartz B, Dowell SF. The common cold - principles of judicious use of antimicrobial agents. Pediatrics 1998;101(1):181-4.

34. Nandimath MK, Ahuja S. Drug prescribing pattern in upper respiratory tract infection in children aged 1 - 14 years. Int J Pharma Bio Sci 2012;3(1):299-308.

35. Joseph N, Bharathi DR, Sreenivasa B, Nataraj GR, George N, Safdar M. Prescribing pattern of drugs in upper respiratory tract infections in pediatric out patients. Int J Contemp Pediatr 2016;3(3):1006-8.

36. Bikash G, Devarsi C, Daisy P, Deka A. Drug prescribing pattern in respiratory tract infection in children aged 1 to 12 years at outpatient department at Silchar Medical College and Hospital, Assam, India. J Pharm Biomed Sci 2016;6(10): 537–45.

37. Park K. Preventive Medicine in Obstetrics, Paediatrics and Geriartics. Park's textbook of Preventive and Social Medicine, 23rd edition, 2015.

38. Sharma S, Agarwal G. A study on drug prescribing pattern in upper respiratory tract infections among children aged 1-12 years. Int J Basic Clin Pharmacol 2016;5(2):406-10.

39. Tiwari P, Ahlawat R, Gupta G. Prescription practice in patients of upper respiratory tract infection at a pediatric outpatient clinic in Punjab. Indian Journal of Pharmacy Practice 2014;7(2):26-32.

40. Kotwani A, Holloway K. Antibiotic prescribing practice for acute, uncomplicated respiratory tract infections in primary care settings in New Delhi, India. Trop Med Int Health 2014;19(7):761-8.

41. Shankar PR, Upadhyay DK, Subish P, Dubey AK, Mishra P. Prescribing patterns among paediatric inpatients in a teaching hospital in western Nepal. Singapore Med J 2006;47(4):261-5.

42. Masavkar SP, Naikwadi AM. Study of incidence of upper respiratory tract infections in urban and rural population. Sch J App Med Sci 2016;4(6C):2023-6.

43. Nash DR, Harman J, Wald ER, Kelleher KJ. Antibiotic prescribing by primary care physicians for children with upper respiratory tract infections. Arch Pediatr Adolesc Med 2002;156(11):1114-9.

44. Wang EE1, Einarson TR, Kellner JD, Conly JM. Antibiotic prescribing for Canadian preschool children: evidence of overprescribing for viral respiratory infections. Clin Infect Dis 1999;29(1):155-60.

45. Gaur AH, Hare ME, Shorr RI. Provider and practice characteristics associated with antibiotic use in children with presumed viral respiratory tract infections. Pediatrics 2005;115(3):635-41.

46. Dawadi S, Rao BS, Khan GM. Pattern of antimicrobial prescription and its cost analysis in respiratory tract infection. Kathmandu

University Journal of Science, Engineering and Technology 2005;1(1):1-9.

47. Alumran A, Hurst C, Xiang-Yu H. Antibiotics Overuse in Children with Upper Respiratory Tract Infections in Saudi Arabia: Risk Factors and Potential Interventions. Clinical Medicine and Diagnostics 2011;1(1):8-16.

48. Oshikoya KA, Chukwura HA. Evaluation of outpatient paediatric drug prescriptions in a teaching hospital in Nigeria for rational prescribing. Paediatr Perinat Drug Ther 2006;7(4):183-8.

49. Razon Y, Ashkenazi S, Cohen A, et al. Effect of educational intervention on antibiotic prescription practices for upper respiratory infections in children: a multicentre study. J Antimicrob Chemother 2005;56(5):937-40.

50. Koch A, Sørensen P, Homøe P, et al. Population-based study of acute respiratory infections in children, Greenland. Emerg Infect Dis 2002;8(6):586–93.

51. Schaad UB, Principi N. The management of recurrent respiratory tract infections in children. Eur Infect Dis 2012;6(2):111-5.

52. de Vries TP, Henning RH, Hogerzeil HV, et al. Impact of a short course in pharmacotherapy for undergraduate medical students: an international randomised controlled study. Lancet 1995;346(8988): 1454-7.